I0696686

WORK HARD
BREATHE &
LET IT ALL OUT

Vulnerability Is Human Not A Weakness

Men's Self Care Guide To A Balanced Life.

By
CYNTHIA LEONARD

All rights reserved.

No part of this publication may be reproduced, distributed or transmitted in any form or by any means, including photocopying, recording or other electronic or mechanical methods, without prior written permission of the publisher, except in the case of brief quotations embodied in critical reviews and certain other non-commercial uses permitted by copyright law.

Copyright © [CYNTHIA LEONARD] 2023

TABLE OF CONTENTS

Dedicated To
ALL MEN OUT THERE

PART 1: THE SILENT STRUGGLE

The "**Silent Struggle**" for men is a term used to describe the challenges and pressures they face in society. Men often face societal expectations, such as being stoic, powerful and the primary source of income, which can make it difficult for them to seek help or express their emotions. This can lead to the concealment of weaknesses or emotions.

Mental health issues, such as depression and anxiety, may arise due to stigma and cultural expectations. Men may also face social isolation, especially as they age, which can negatively impact their mental and emotional health. Navigating relationships can be challenging, especially when it comes to showing vulnerability and expressing feelings.

Fatherhood demands and obligations can also make it difficult for men to balance work, family and personal life. Pressure to succeed in their careers can lead to stress, burnout, and a commitment to work that compromises their overall wellbeing.

Physical health issues may arise due to men's reluctance to use preventative healthcare or seek medical treatment, potentially leading to unrecognised or untreated health problems. Addiction and substance misuse may also be a concern for many men.

Identity and self-discovery are also significant challenges faced by men, as they struggle to balance societal expectations with their genuine selves. Stereotyping and discrimination based on gender can negatively impact their prospects and overall well-being.

Importance Of This Journey

Men's self-care is an essential component of overall wellness and should be embraced as a journey for a number of reasons:

Men's mental health may be greatly enhanced by practising self-care. It enables men to deal with their emotions, lower their stress levels and avoid burnout. Better mental toughness and the capacity to successfully navigate the obstacles of life may result from this.

Physical Health: Taking care of one's physical health includes getting regular exercise, eating a balanced diet and getting enough sleep. These behaviours may improve physical health, reduce the risk of chronic illnesses, and lengthen life expectancy.

Emotional Well-Being: Self-care enables men to better understand and connect with their emotions. This may result in happier relationships, better communication abilities and a higher level of empathy and comprehension.

Reduced Toxic Masculinity: Men are often socialised to repress their feelings and adhere to strict gender standards. Self-care activities may support the development of healthy masculine expressions and assist in eradicating these negative behaviours.

Increased Productivity: Self-care may result in improved productivity, attention, and creativity. Men are better able to function successfully in both their personal and professional life when they take time to relax and recharge.

Relationships: Self-care techniques that are wholesome may enhance relationships. When men put their health first, they may be more attentive and helpful as friends, dads and spouses.

Prevention of drug addiction: Practising self-care might lessen the propensity to adopt hazardous coping strategies, such as drug addiction, while handling stress or emotional challenges.

Self-Awareness: Taking care of oneself promotes introspection and self-awareness. Men who are able to better understand their wants, beliefs and ambitions live lives that are more meaningful and gratifying. By taking care of themselves, men may serve as great role models for future generations. In the future, this may encourage healthy attitudes towards self-care and interrupt the cycle of toxic masculinity.

Long-Term Happiness: In the end, self-care helps people be happy and satisfied with their lives in the long run. Men who put their health first are more likely to enjoy happy lives and have optimistic outlooks on the future.

The notion of self-care is not universal. Men should look into and choose self-care techniques that speak to them individually, whether it's writing, meditation, spending time in nature, going to counselling or indulging in interests and hobbies. Self-care is a process that never ends and should be seen as an investment in one's overall wellbeing.

PART 2: THE HARDWORKING MAN

<u>Work Ethic</u>

A set of morals and beliefs that place a high priority on perseverance, commitment and hard effort in order to fulfil one's obligations is known as a strong work ethic. It entails a methodical approach to activities and a readiness to put up the necessary effort to succeed at one's profession.

The following are some crucial elements of the work ethic:

Strong work ethics are shown by those who are committed to their job and take their obligations seriously. They are dedicated to giving every work they take on their all.

Reliability: People with a good work ethic are seen as being reliable. They are trustworthy and reliable, arriving on time and meeting deadlines.

Persistence in the face of difficulties is a key component of a strong work ethic. Those with a strong work ethic keep working hard to overcome challenges or setbacks, even in the face of them.

Efficiency: Having a good work ethic entails using both effort and intelligence. The key ingredients are effective work practises and time management abilities.

Self-control: Those with strong work ethics possess a high level of self-control. They are able to be productive because they can maintain their attention and keep away from outside distractions.

Professionalism is often correlated with a strong work ethic. This entails keeping a cheerful outlook, exhibiting respect for coworkers and clients and upholding moral principles.

Improvement through Time: People with excellent work ethics are often motivated to advance both personally and professionally. They look for chances to learn and develop.

Accountability: Individuals with a strong work ethic accept ownership of their decisions and results. They don't provide justifications or assign responsibility for their mistakes.

A strong work ethic places an emphasis on working hard, but it also understands the need of maintaining a good work-life balance. Workplace burnout is not a viable strategy.

High expectations: People with good work ethics often set high criteria for themselves and push themselves to do their best job.

Successful people frequently have good work ethics because they are more productive, perform better at their jobs and have more opportunity to progress their careers. It's a desirable quality in many spheres of life, including the job, academia and extracurricular activities. To prevent working too much or ignoring other facets of life, it's crucial to find a balance.

<u>**Physical And Mental Toll**</u>

Due to their passion and commitment to their profession, hard working people *(regardless of gender)* often experience tremendous physical and mental tolls.

Hardworking males may put in long hours, do physically taxing duties and have little downtime. This may result in exhaustion, muscular aches and a compromised immune system. Chronic health problems including hypertension, obesity or cardiac difficulties might develop as a consequence of time.

Excessive levels of stress and anxiety may result from the pressure to satisfy work-related objectives, deadlines and expectations. Long-term mental health consequences of this stress may include depression, anxiety disorders or burnout, among other mental health issues. It might be difficult for motivated people to maintain a positive work-life balance. Isolation, strained family dynamics, and a worse quality of life may result from disregarding personal time, relationships and interests.

Stress from the workplace and long hours might interfere with sleep cycles. Lack of sleep may have a significant negative effect on one's physical and mental health, affecting one's ability to think clearly, control their emotions and feel generally well, while busy schedules might prevent hardworking people from prioritising routine medical checkups or recognising the signs of sickness. Health problems may take longer to diagnose and cure as a consequence.

To deal with the stress and strain of their jobs, some people abuse drugs or alcohol. This may worsen mental health difficulties and cause addiction problems.

Hardworking men may find it difficult to manage their personal and professional life, which may lead to strained relationships with spouses, kids or other family members. Feelings of guilt, frustration and loneliness may result from this.

Busy people could forget to engage in self-care activities like exercise, a balanced diet and downtime. Over time, this may worsen problems with one's physical and mental health. Despite their commitment, diligent men may feel decreasing job satisfaction as a consequence of the toll on their physical and mental health. Disillusionment and a sense of futility may result from this.

Increased Burnout Risk is a condition marked by emotional tiredness, poor performance and cynicism. It may be brought on by extended periods of hard labour. Recovery often requires lengthy absences from work and supportive mental health services.

For those who put in a lot of effort, it's important to recognise the symptoms of physical and emotional exhaustion and practise self-care, also getting help when you need it is a high priority. The promotion of a positive workplace culture that prioritises work-life balance and staff wellbeing is within the purview of employers.

Recognizing The Need For Change

A dedicated person who has consistently worked hard but finds their current situation unfulfilling may recognize the need for change. This may be due to factors such as burnout, a desire for personal development, changes in their industry or circumstances. Some potential responses include adjusting stress levels, work-life balance and self-care priorities.

Career change may be necessary if the person becomes bored or disillusioned after working in the same field for a long time. This could involve exploring other employment options, learning new skills, or starting a new hobby. Adapting to market changes, such as technological advancements or customer preferences, may also be necessary.

Personal development may involve setting new goals, seeking educational opportunities or accepting more challenging challenges. Relationships may also need change, as the individual may realise that their social networks are no longer beneficial.

The environment may also need to be considered, as relocating to a different area or changing their office may increase productivity and well-being. Financial planning may also need to be adjusted to ensure a brighter future by altering spending patterns, budgeting, or investment plans.

Understanding that change is necessary is often the first step towards both personal and professional development. Once this realisation happens, it's important for the person to plan a strategy, establish clear objectives and take concrete measures to make the required adjustments in their life. Change may be difficult, but over time it can also result in greater achievement, satisfaction and success.

PART 3: EMBRACING SELF-CARE

Redefining Self-Care For Men

In order to dispel gender norms and advance everyone's holistic wellbeing, men's self-care has to be redefined. Men have traditionally been discouraged from publicly discussing or prioritising self-care due to traditional conceptions of masculinity, but this is changing as society realises the need of mental and emotional health for all people, regardless of gender.

Men might redefine self-care in the following ways:

- Encourage men to communicate their feelings honestly and to ask for help when they need it. This may include discussing their emotions, thoughts and worries with friends, family or a therapist.

- Men's self-care practices should include frequent exercise, a healthy diet and enough rest. Maintaining one's physical health is an important part of practising self-care since it is directly related to maintaining one's mental health.

- The importance of mental health is equal to that of physical health. Encourage males to get medical attention for mental health conditions such stress, anxiety or depression. Destigmatize counselling and therapy.

- Promote healthy connections with your friends and romantic partners. Encourage emotional connection and honest conversation since they are crucial for wellbeing.

- Promote men's participation in their hobbies and interests. Self-care may be as simple as participating in things that one is enthusiastic about, which can assist to lower stress and increase overall contentment.

- Assist men in balancing their personal and professional life. Prioritising downtime and leisure activities is crucial since working too much might result in burnout.

- Promote mindfulness techniques and meditation as methods for reducing stress and enhancing mental clarity. These routines may support guys in being steady and concentrated.

- Men should be taught the value of having self-compassion. Self-criticism may be detrimental and it's OK to make errors and have shortcomings. Promote self-acceptance and compassion to yourself.

- ***Community and Support Networks:*** It's important to have a reliable support system. Men should be aware that they may turn to friends and relatives for support or just someone to chat to.

- Encourage frequent medical checkups to keep an eye on your physical wellness. Prevention is often simpler and more efficient than addressing health issues after they have gotten out of hand.

- Be aware of cultural differences in self-care across all origins and cultures. Embrace one's cultural background while promoting self-care while respecting individual preferences and practices.

- Confront gender preconceptions and conventional gender norms that may prevent males from engaging in self-care. Men should feel unrestricted in their exploration of hobbies and customs traditionally associated with femininity.

- Encourage males to learn about and practise self-care. It could be good to provide information since many people might not be acquainted with the idea or its advantages.

- By publicly expressing their personal self-care routines, men in leadership roles may serve as role models and show that doing so is a sign of strength rather than weakness.

Men's self-care is being redefined by fostering an environment of acceptance, help and emotional intelligence. We can help create healthier, happier people and communities by encouraging men to put their physical, emotional and mental well-being first.

Physical Well-Being

Men's physical well-being is taking care of your body via a variety
of healthy lifestyle choices, such as food, exercise, routine
checkups with the doctor and stress management. *Here are some
important factors to think about:*

Nutrition and Diet:

- Eat a varied diet that contains whole grains, lean proteins,
  fresh fruits and vegetables and healthy fats.

- Limit your consumption of processed meals, sweet
  beverages, and a lot of red meat.

- Drink a lot of water throughout the day to stay hydrated.

Regular Workouts:

- Exercise regularly, incorporating both strength training
  (lifting weights or bodyweight exercises) and aerobic activities
  (such as jogging or cycling).

- As well as muscle-strengthening exercises on two or more
  days each week, aim for at least 150 minutes of
  moderate-intensity aerobic activity or 75 minutes of
  vigorous-intensity aerobic exercise each week.

Sleep:

- Make obtaining 7-9 hours of good sleep each night a
  priority. The key to general health and wellbeing is getting
  enough sleep.

Stress Reduction:

- To successfully manage stress, try stress-reduction exercises
  like yoga, deep breathing, meditation or mindfulness.

- Regular medical examinations

- To get frequent checkups and screenings, see your doctor.
  This may aid in early health problem detection and
  treatment.

Heart Wellness:

- Pay close attention to your heart health. This entails
  keeping an eye on cholesterol and blood pressure levels as
  well as adopting preventative measures against heart
  disease.

Mental Wellness:

- Make sure your mental health is taken care of by getting
  help when you need it. The importance of mental and
  physical wellness is equal.

Avoid Smoking and Drink in moderation:

If you do drink, exercise moderation. Avoid using tobacco in any manner, including smoking.

Keeping a Healthy Weight in Mind:

Using a mix of food and exercise, reach and maintain a healthy body weight. If you need advice, speak with a medical expert.

Hygiene:

Use proper personal hygiene, such as taking frequent showers, taking care of your teeth and grooming.

Routine Physical Examinations:

- Check your body often for changes, such as skin anomalies or strange lumps, and contact a doctor right once if you see anything unsettling.

Safety:

To avoid mishaps and injuries, use vigilance at work and during leisure activities.

Social Networking:

Maintain positive relationships with friends and family as well as good social ties. Having a solid support system may improve your wellbeing as a whole.

Exercise and Nutrition

Men's self-care includes a variety of activities that support their emotional, mental, and physical well. Men's self-care must include both exercise and diet since they are so important for preserving general health and vigour.

Exercise:

Cardiovascular Health: Cardiovascular health may be improved by regular activity, such as brisk walking, running, cycling or swimming. It improves heart health, brings down blood pressure, and decreases the risk of heart attack and stroke.

Weight control: By burning calories and boosting metabolic rate, exercise may help with weight management. For general health, it's essential to maintain a healthy weight.

Muscle Strength: Workouts for building and maintaining muscle mass include bodyweight workouts or weightlifting. This may help everyday tasks and increase physical strength.

Bone Health: Weight-bearing activities like strength training and jogging help to maintain bone health and may lower the risk of osteoporosis.

Exercise is a great way to reduce stress naturally. Endorphins, mood-boosting chemicals that lessen tension and anxiety, are released as a result of it.

Improved Sleep: Regular exercise may improve the quantity and quality of sleep as well as assist treat sleep problems including insomnia.

Nutrition:

Diet: An ideal diet for men's self-care should include a mix of fruits, vegetables, lean meats, whole grains and healthy fats. This gives the body the nutrition it needs for maximum performance. Nutritionally sound eating is essential for keeping a healthy weight. Monitoring portion sizes and eating nutrient-dense meals may help with weight management.

Energy Levels: Eating consistent, wholesome meals and snacks throughout the day may help stabilise energy levels, decreasing weariness and boosting productivity.

Disease Prevention: A nutritious diet helps lower the chance of developing chronic conditions including diabetes, heart disease and certain types of cancer.

Nutrition has a part in one's mental wellness. For instance, omega-3 fatty acids, which are present in fatty fish, may have mood-enhancing properties. Avoiding excessive amounts of coffee and sweets may also help control anxiety and mood swings.

Hydration: It's important to maintain a healthy level of hydration. Enough water consumption aids in digestion, controls body temperature and maintains healthy skin and organs.

Men's self-care requires incorporating exercise and healthy eating into everyday routines. A personalised plan that is in line with each person's unique requirements and objectives for their health should be developed after consultation with a qualified dietician or healthcare expert. A healthy lifestyle may be attained and maintained over the long term with progressive lifestyle modifications and the formulation of attainable objectives.

Sleep And Rest

Self-care is essential for both men and women, as it provides numerous emotional, mental and physical benefits. To ensure good self-care, it is crucial to prioritise sleep and relaxation.

Men should aim for 7-9 hours of restful sleep per night, establish a peaceful bedtime routine and avoid stimulating activities like watching TV or using electronic devices.

Ensure a comfortable sleeping environment by making the bedroom sleep-friendly, adjusting the temperature and reducing noise and light.

Limit alcohol and caffeine intake, regular physical activity and be mindful of food choices before bed. Manage stress by practising relaxation exercises like progressive muscle relaxation, deep breathing or meditation.

Limit screen time by using blue light-blocking eyewear or adding blue light filters to your devices.

Avoid napping, as taking long or inconsistent naps throughout the day can interfere with sleep patterns at night. Consult a medical expert if you frequently experience sleep problems like insomnia or sleep apnea for advice, identifying underlying issues and suggesting viable therapies.

Maintain hydration by limiting fluid consumption close to bedtime and avoiding distractions like office supplies or computer devices.

Maintain a consistent sleep schedule by going to bed and waking at the same times every day, even on weekends. Pay attention to your body's cues and take short breaks or fast sleep if necessary. Seek social support to discuss your self-care goals with friends or others in your support system.

Prioritising your well-being, including sleep and relaxation, is essential for maintaining excellent physical and mental health. By following these tips, men can improve their overall well-being.

Mental And Emotional Well-Being

Everyone, especially males, needs to be in good mental and emotional health. Unfortunately, males often find it difficult to freely discuss their mental and emotional health because of cultural norms and preconceptions. However, in order to live a happy and balanced life, it's essential to put mental and emotional health first.

Men's mental and emotional wellbeing is crucial for their overall well-being. It is essential to express your feelings, whether happy or negative, to prevent stress and worsen mental health conditions.

Seeking support from close friends, family or a therapist is also recommended. Physical well-being, such as regular exercise, a balanced diet and adequate sleep, can significantly impact mental health. Mindfulness and meditation can help lower stress levels and enhance emotional resilience.

Building strong social ties can also benefit mental health. Spending time with loved ones and friends can strengthen bonds. Setting achievable goals for personal and professional lives can improve overall wellbeing and self-worth. Managing stress through healthy methods like meditation, hobbies or creative pursuits can also help.

Self-compassion can reduce emotional suffering and boost self-esteem.

Limiting substance use is crucial to prevent worsening mental health problems. If you suspect substance misuse, seek treatment. Seeking expert advice from therapists, counsellors or other mental health experts can provide valuable support.

Educating yourself about emotional and mental wellness is essential for maintaining mental health. Challenging gender preconceptions can also deter men from seeking help or expressing their feelings. Recognizing that it is okay to express weakness and seek help is crucial for maintaining mental and emotional well-being.

Being mentally and emotionally healthy requires continual effort. Although difficulties are common, you can maintain and even enhance your mental and emotional health with the correct resources and assistance. Never be afraid to ask for assistance when you need it and place a high priority on self-care as a vital component of your general well-being.

<u>Stress Management</u>

Effective stress management is crucial for everyone, but men may face unique challenges and cultural pressures that may affect their handling of stress. Men can benefit from recognizing and addressing stress, expressing their emotions to loved ones and practising relaxation techniques like progressive muscle relaxation, deep breathing exercises and meditation.

Creating reasonable expectations and maintaining a balanced diet, sleep and limiting alcohol and caffeine consumption can help manage stress.

Time management strategies can help organise obligations and chores, while seeking professional help when necessary can enhance mental health and learn stress management techniques.

Joining a support group can also be a powerful stress-reduction tool, as it allows individuals to spend time with loved ones and friends who can help them feel better.

Finding hobbies and interests outside of work can also help relax and unwind. Mindfulness meditation can help control stress by embracing emotions without judgement.

Limiting technology and screen time can also help manage stress. It's important to remember that managing stress is a personal process and it's essential to test out various methods and ideas to find the one that works best for each individual.

Meditation And Mindfulness

For men's self-care, mindfulness and meditation are effective strategies. They may aid in stress reduction, mental wellness, self-awareness enhancement and emotional regulation promotion.

Here are some ideas and information regarding how guys might include mindfulness and meditation in their self-care practises:

Know the advantages:

- Men may manage their stress, anxiety and depression with the use of mindfulness and meditation.

- They raise productivity by sharpening attention and concentration.

- Better relationships may result from these techniques' promotion of emotional intelligence and self-awareness.

- They support improved rest and general physical wellbeing.

Begin Small:

- Each day, start with only a few minutes of meditation, then as you become more comfortable, extend it.

- To get you started, you may select videos or applications that provide guided meditation.

Pick a Relaxing Location:

- Find a spot to meditate that is peaceful and distraction-free.

- Use a chair or a cushion for more comfort.

Breathing Consciously:

- Watch your breath as it comes and passes. Keep your focus on your chest's ups and downs as well as the feeling of breath at your nostrils.

- Bring your focus back to your breath softly and without judgement when your mind wanders *(which it will)*.

The Body Scan:

- By consciously scanning your body, you may practise mindfulness by noticing any tension or discomfort.

- It's a powerful method for releasing physical stress and raising your awareness of your body's requirements.

Mindfulness Practises:

You may integrate awareness into regular tasks; formal meditation is not required. Consider how your meal tastes and feels while you consume. Pay attention to each step you take while you walk.

Achieving Consistency:

- Consistency is crucial with any self-care routine. Try to create a daily schedule.

- If you skip a day, simply get back on track the next day.

Find Assistance:

- If you want to meet others who share your interests, think about joining a meditation or mindfulness group, either in person or online.

- A therapist or counsellor who focuses on mindfulness-based treatments is another resource you may use.

Follow Your Needs:

There are several approaches to men's self-care. Find what works best for you by experimenting with various mindfulness and meditation practices.

Realistic Goal Setting:

Expecting quick outcomes is unrealistic. Be patient with yourself since the advantages of mindfulness and meditation may not become obvious right away.

Keep in mind that mindfulness and meditation are all about accepting yourself as you are and being present in the moment. They may be useful self-care methods that can strengthen your emotional stability, increase your emotional resilience and improve your ability to deal with the stresses of everyday life.

Hobbies And Recreation

For everyone, even males, self-care is essential. The promotion of physical and mental well-being is greatly aided by hobbies and recreational activities. Stress reduction, mood enhancement and general quality of life may all be benefited by engaging in enjoyable activities.

Exercise is important for sustaining excellent health on a regular basis. Exercise is a terrific method to lower stress, build confidence and remain in shape, whether you're working out at the gym, cycling, jogging, playing sports or doing yoga.

Camping and hiking: Being outdoors may be quite soothing. You may escape the rigours of everyday life, take in fresh air and establish a connection with nature by hiking and camping.

Fishing is a tranquil and calming hobby. It offers the chance to unwind by the sea, have some alone time or socialise with friends, and maybe even catch supper.

Cooking and grilling: Making and cooking meals on a grill or hob may be a fun and creative activity. An enjoyable and soothing experience may result from experimenting with different recipes and cooking methods.

Music is a wonderful way to relax and express yourself, whether you play an instrument or just listen to it. Your mood and stress levels may both be enhanced by playing music or listening to your favourite songs.

Reading: Reading is a great way to relax, learn new things, and escape into other realms. Whether it's non-fiction, fiction or periodicals, discovering a good book may be a source of solace and intellectual stimulation.

You may express your creativity and capture memories via **Photography**. It may be a thrilling experience to discover new locations to snap pictures.

Gardening: Spending time in the garden not only provides enjoyment and productivity, but it also helps you become closer to nature. It's relaxing and peaceful to take care of plants.

Self-Defense and Martial Arts Training: Learning self-defence or martial arts may increase self-assurance, enhance physical fitness and impart useful skills for personal protection.

Playing games: Playing board games or video games may be a relaxing way to pass the time. To maintain a good balance, just practise moderation.

DIY projects are satisfying ways to spend your time. Building, making, or remodelling are examples. Your feeling of achievement is increased and your creativity is released when you finish DIY tasks.

Giving back to your community by volunteering may be a rewarding and worthwhile way to spend your time. It may enhance your mental health and give you a feeling of purpose.

PART 4: THE POWER OF CONNECTION

Men And Loneliness

In recent years, there has been an uptick in discussion about men and loneliness. Despite the fact that loneliness is a widespread problem that may affect anybody, regardless of gender, men may find it more difficult to face and communicate their loneliness due to certain social and cultural circumstances.

Here are some important factors to think about:

Social Expectations: Men are often expected to be stoic, self-sufficient, and emotionally repressed by traditional cultural conventions. These standards may deter males from openly expressing their loneliness or asking for emotional help.

Stigma: Men who confess to being lonely or who display vulnerability may be subject to stigma. Some guys may be afraid of coming out as weak or less manly if they admit to feeling lonely.

Lack of Social Support: Men may experience emotions of loneliness since their social networks may be less than those of women. An emphasis on work or a profession, a reluctance to reach out to others, or social expectations that males should have fewer personal connections are some possible causes of this.

Relationship Patterns: Some men could depend heavily on their romantic partner for emotional support, which can be troublesome if the relationship fails or if they don't have a solid support structure outside of their spouse.

Mental Health: Depression and anxiety are two mental health conditions that are directly correlated with loneliness. Men may be less inclined to seek professional assistance for mental health issues, which makes them feel even more alone.

Communication: Men and women may communicate in different ways, which may cause misunderstandings in relationships and exacerbate feelings of loneliness. Men may be more apt to look for answers to issues than to express their feelings.

Men's Loneliness need a Diverse Strategy:

- Encourage guys to speak about their sentiments openly and express their emotions without fear of being judged. The stigma attached to vulnerability may be lessened by creating a secure environment for free conversation.

- It is important to encourage men to create and maintain a variety of social support systems, including those with friends, family, and peers.

- Raise awareness of the value of mental health and the services that are available in this area. Encourage men to get assistance from a professional if they need it.

- Create a greater understanding of how gender norms and cultural expectations may make males feel lonely. Dispel these myths and support broader, more nimble notions of masculinity.

- Support and take part in community initiatives aimed at reducing loneliness and isolation, especially among males.

It's important to understand that loneliness is a common human emotion and that in order to address it, gender-related obstacles must be removed in order to promote a more accepting and compassionate society in which everyone feels free to ask for assistance when they need it.

Building Supportive Relationships

For both personal and professional well-being, developing supportive connections is crucial. Supportive relationships provide a feeling of community, trust and security by offering emotional, social and even practical aid when required.

Some guidelines for creating and sustaining helpful relationships:

Communication that works:

Avoid interrupting people while paying attention to what they are saying. Recognise their emotions and worries and provide empathy.

Honesty and respect should be used while expressing your demands. Understanding is enhanced through direct and open conversation.

Understanding and Compassion:

Make an effort to comprehend the thoughts and feelings of others. A higher degree of connection with others is made possible through empathy. Keep your opinions and presumptions about their experiences to yourself.

Integrity and Trust:

Be dependable by maintaining your word and acting in a consistent manner. Any connection that is helpful must be built on trust, the key is dependability. People should trust that they may turn to you for assistance.

Make yourself Available:

Schedule time for your social life. Prioritise family time even when you have a hectic schedule. Whether it's at a happy occasion or a trying one, be there when they need you.

Offer Aid and Assistance:

When you see someone suffering, be quick to offer support. Inform them that you are ready to assist and be considerate of their requirements and preferences. Even if someone doesn't want aid, they may nevertheless value the knowledge that it is accessible.

Observe Boundaries:

Recognise and honour others' privacy limits. As required, give them some room. Don't push them to provide or receive more help than they are willing to.

Good Interactions:

When you're together, cultivate a friendly and encouraging environment. Exchange amusement, wisdom and fun.
Join in the celebration of your successes and accomplishments.

Resolving Disputes:

Any partnership will always have conflicts. Be patient and ready to work things out when you talk to them. Instead of lingering on the issue, concentrate on finding solutions.

Self-Care:

Maintaining helpful relationships requires taking care of oneself. If you're mentally or emotionally spent, you can't help people very well. Put your personal wants in perspective with those of your loved ones.

Be Apologetic and Forgiving:

When you mess up or accidentally harm someone, honestly apologise. Also be ready to pardon people when they wrong you or do you harm. Relationships may suffer from holding grudges.

Honour Differences:

Respect each person's individuality and embrace variety in your life. Relationships may become stronger when differences are recognised.

Commitment Over Time:

It takes time to develop a supporting network. Maintaining these relationships over time will need patience and commitment.

Relations with Colleagues:

Incorporate these ideas into your work life as well. A career that is more enjoyable and productive might result from developing helpful connections at work.

Keep in mind that connections of support are mutually beneficial. Maintaining and developing them requires participation from both sides. Building these connections requires time and effort, but the benefits in terms of mental health and a solid support network are well worth it.

The Role Of Friendships

Friendships are crucial for men's overall health and self-care. They offer a secure environment for men to express their feelings and vulnerability, reducing stress and enhancing emotional health.

Spending time with friends can lower stress levels by encouraging bonding and releasing the stress hormone cortisol.

Strong friendships are linked to improved mental health outcomes, especially for men struggling with anxiety, depression and other mental health issues.

Friendships also provide a sense of community and belonging, increasing one's sense of value and self-worth. They can serve as a helpful coping strategy during trying times, providing guidance, empathy and a listening ear. Physical well-being can be maintained through participation in physical activities with friends, inspiring active lifestyles and good habits.

Friendships also offer opportunities for social skill development and improvement, such as communication, conflict resolution and empathy.

Enjoyment and fun are essential components of self-care, increasing overall happiness and life satisfaction.

Accountability is another benefit of friendships. Having friends who share similar goals can inspire and encourage men in maintaining their self-care practices and objectives.

Strong social ties, especially friendships, have been linked to a longer lifetime, helping men overcome life's problems and maintain a happier, more fulfilled life.

Men should prioritise and take care of their friendships as part of their self-care regimen. The creation and maintenance of these relationships may enhance one's physical, mental and emotional health. Men should also understand that asking for aid and support from friends is an important part of self-care and is a show of strength, not weakness.

<u>**Seeking Professional Help**</u>

Seeking professional help for mental health issues is important for men, as it is an indication of strength rather than weakness.

It is essential to normalise the concept of seeking help and choose the correct professional, considering factors such as gender, cultural acuity and treatment style. Open communication with your therapist or counsellor is essential, as it allows you to voice your concerns and desired outcomes from treatment.

Consistency in treatment is paramount, as real transformation often requires time and effort. Group therapy offers a safe space for males to interact with others going through similar struggles, removing feelings of isolation.

Medication may be included in treatment strategies when necessary, but it is important to consult a psychiatrist to determine if it is right for you.

Body health is another important aspect of self-care, involving regular exercise, a healthy diet and sufficient sleep. Managing stress through techniques like yoga, deep breathing, mindfulness and meditation can ease tension and enhance mental clarity.

Establishing limits helps avoid burnout and maintain a good work-life balance. Learning when to say no is also essential.

Lean on support systems, including friends, family and support groups, to foster emotional comfort and a sense of community. Regular self-reflection can help identify triggers, trends and potential development areas.

Don't wait until problems become too difficult to seek help; get treatment immediately if you detect persistent changes in mood, behaviour or mental health. Early intervention often yields better results.

A key stage in the self-care process is to seek professional assistance. Doing so may result in better mental and emotional health as well as a more satisfying existence.

PART 5: UNMASKING YOUR EMOTIONS

<u>Stigma Around Male Emotions</u>

The social and cultural expectations and prejudices that sometimes prevent men and boys from freely expressing their feelings are referred to as the stigma surrounding masculine emotions.

Both people and society as a whole may suffer negative effects as a result of this stigma.

Traditional Gender Roles: There are long-standing gender roles in many countries that specify how men and women should act. Men are often seen as austere, powerful and emotionless, while women are viewed as caring and expressive. Because of these expectations, males may find it challenging to express their sensitivity or ask for emotional help.

The term "toxic masculinity" refers to detrimental societal expectations and norms connected to conventional masculinity. It often encourages violence, the repression of emotions and the notion that showing emotion is a sign of weakness. Men may worry about being criticised or mocked for displaying vulnerability as a result, which may lead to a stigma around masculine emotions.

Mental Health: The stigma associated with masculine emotions may seriously affect men's mental health. Men's resistance to seeking support or expressing their emotions might result in untreated mental health conditions including depression and anxiety. In certain communities, this may lead to increased rates of suicide among males.

A lack of honest emotional expression may cause problems in interpersonal bonds. Men who are emotionally distant may find it difficult to connect with their partners, families and friends. This may result in miscommunications and make it challenging to keep up positive connections.

Workplace: In certain workplaces, men's emotions are stigmatised and it is expected that they always present as powerful and collected. Men may find it difficult to confront workplace stress, discrimination or harassment because of this. It could also deter them from requesting flexible work schedules or parental leave to assist their families.

Changing Attitudes: Thankfully, perceptions of masculine emotions are evolving throughout time. To combat stereotypes and advance healthy forms of masculinity, a variety of advocacy groups, mental health organisations and individuals are at work. Men's feelings are being spoken more openly as a result of movements like ***#MeToo*** and growing mental health awareness.

Media Representation: The media significantly influences cultural views and conventions. The stigma associated with masculine emotions may be fought by presenting a larger variety of emotionally expressive and sensitive male characters.
By encouraging emotional intelligence and educating kids and young people that it's appropriate for boys and men to express their emotions and seek assistance when they need it, schools and educational institutions may play a critical part in removing this stigma.

The stigma associated with masculine emotions is a complicated problem with roots in society and cultural conventions. For the sake of advancing mental health and more satisfying interpersonal connections in society, it is essential to challenge these prejudices and promote free and healthy emotional expression for everyone, regardless of gender.

Impact Of Suppressing Emotions

Suppressing feelings negatively affects men's self-care and general wellbeing. Although society often pushes males to remain stoic and suppress their emotions, this may have a number of detrimental effects.

- Suppressing feelings might result in an increase in stress. When emotions are suppressed, the body's stress response is triggered, which may have long-term negative effects on health, such as cardiovascular issues and weakened immune system.

- Conditions like anxiety and depression may develop or worsen as a result of suppressing emotions. To preserve excellent mental health, it's important to recognise and express emotions.

- Human connection is mostly based on emotions. It may be challenging to establish and sustain meaningful connections if they are suppressed. Keeping feelings within might lead to angry or frustrated outbursts that harm relationships.

- Suppression of emotions might limit self-awareness and personal development. Insights into one's ideas, feelings and wants may be gained through one's emotions. Ignoring them might hinder one's growth and ability to progress.

- Consistent emotional repression has been associated with a number of physical health difficulties, such as headaches, digestive problems and sleep disorders. These physical

symptoms may also have an adverse effect on general
health.

- Some men may adopt unhealthy strategies to cope with
  repressed emotions, such as drug misuse or binge eating,
  which may result in addiction and health issues.

Encouragement of emotional expression and the creation of
environments where men feel comfortable talking about their
emotions are mandatory for enhancing men's self-care and
wellbeing.

Men should be educated that asking for assistance from friends,
family or mental health experts when necessary is not a sign of
weakness. Men may improve their emotional awareness and
management by engaging in mindfulness practises like journaling
and meditation.

Learning To Identify And Express Feelings

Emotional health is crucial for overall well-being and men should
practise self-care to recognize and express their emotions. Men can
do this by practising self-awareness, normalising emotions, talking
to a reliable person, learning emotional vocabulary, using
mindfulness practices like meditation and deep breathing,
consulting a mental health expert if struggling with emotions or
dealing with chronic mental health problems and reflecting on
one's sentiments and reasons behind them.

Avoid self-criticism and focus on self-compassion, as it is essential
to avoid making errors and feeling vulnerable. Engage in activities
that enhance emotional health, such as creative endeavours,
music, physical activity or being outside. Set boundaries in

relationships and everyday life, ensuring that you prioritise your own emotional needs.

Defy outdated ideas about masculinity that may limit emotional expressiveness and recognize that being in touch with your emotions indicates strength rather than weakness. Encourage honest discussions about feelings with friends, family and classmates to support others and foster a more emotionally healthy community.

Developing the ability to recognize and communicate emotions is a lifelong process that can result in better mental and emotional health, greater interpersonal bonds and a more rewarding existence.

It is important to take care of your mental wellbeing, not be too harsh on yourself and ask for assistance when needed. By doing so, men can improve their overall well-being and contribute to a healthier and happier life.

Tools And Techniques For Healthy Expression

Men may encourage healthy self-expression and self-care by using the following tools and techniques:

- Begin with recognising that it's OK to feel and express emotions. Avoid holding your emotions within.

- Reduce stress and raise your emotional awareness by engaging in mindfulness and meditation.

- Regular exercise is healthy for your body as well as your mind. Make a habit of doing a physical exercise you like.

- Be sure you eat a balanced diet, receive the right nutrients and drink enough water.

- Keep a diary of your thoughts and emotions to better understand how you're feeling.

- Discuss your feelings with a trusted person. Sharing your worries and experiences might help you feel better and get support.

- Take up creative pursuits like drawing, writing, playing an instrument or any other kind of artistic expression.

- Stress relief and emotional regulation may both be accomplished via creativity.

- Create and sustain enduring bonds with your friends, family, and partners. Open dialogue is essential.

- If you're having trouble with your relationships or with emotional difficulties, get expert assistance.

- Study stress-reduction methods including yoga, progressive muscle relaxation and deep breathing.

- Set aside time for leisurely pursuits and rest.

- Consider your objectives, principles and desires carefully. Ask yourself often whether your life is in line with these values.

- Despite how modest they may appear, set attainable objectives and acknowledge your successes.

- Do not be reluctant to seek assistance from a therapist, counsellor, or support group if you are struggling with intense emotions, mental health problems or addiction.

Getting help from a professional is nothing to be ashamed of and facing your difficulties head-on is a show of courage.

- Pay attention to the amount of time you spend on devices and social media. A lot of screen time might be bad for your mental health.

- Establish a self-care regimen that includes relaxing activities that you love doing.

- Place self-care on the same level of importance as other responsibilities in your everyday life.

- Maintain your learning and challenge yourself. Personal development may be immensely rewarding. Expand your horizons by reading books, enrolling in classes or taking up new activities.

- Join organisations or networks for guys that promote candid discussion about self-care and mental health. Also surround yourself with understanding and supporting individuals.

PART 6: THE ART OF COMMUNICATION

<u>Effective Communication</u>

A key component of men's self-care is effective communication since it not only strengthens bonds between people but also promotes mental and emotional health. As part of their self-care regimen, men might benefit from the following advice on how to communicate effectively:

Active Listening: Pay close attention to what others are saying. Avoid interjecting and concentrate on comprehending their viewpoint rather than planning your reaction.

Don't Suppress Your Feelings or Thoughts: Express yourself. Share your feelings and ideas with someone you can trust, such as a friend, relative or therapist.

Use "I" phrases: To prevent blaming or accusing, use "I" phrases when expressing your thoughts or worries. Instead of saying "You always make me feel...", for instance, use "I feel hurt when..."

Try to comprehend the sentiments and perspective of the other person by practising empathy. Conflict resolution and the development of healthier relationships may both benefit from empathy.

Be Aware of Nonverbal Communication: Your body language, expressions on your face, and tone of voice may say just as much as, if not more, than what you say. Make sure your nonverbal clues support the message you want to convey by being aware of them.

Ask Open-Ended Questions: Promote candid communication by posing inquiries that call for more information than a straightforward "yes" or "no" response. Deeper talks may result from this.

Keep Calm: When presented with challenging talks, refrain from responding rashly. Before answering, take a moment to centre yourself. This may help to avoid misunderstandings and pointless disputes.

Practise Conflict Resolution: Acquire the skills necessary to settle disputes amicably. Avoid personal attacks and instead concentrate on the current problem. Explore areas of agreement and compromise.

Encourage people to provide feedback on your communication style by asking for it. Finding opportunities for development is made easier with constructive criticism.

Use Technology Wisely: In the digital environment we live in, be aware of how technology might impact your ability to communicate. In order to offer your complete attention to the person you are conversing with, put your gadgets aside during significant talks.

Set Limits: Specify your own limits clearly and let others know about them. This aids in stress reduction and expectation management.

Consider your own communication styles by pausing to think about them. Determine the areas where you may need some improvement and focus on them. If you have persistent communication difficulties or unresolved concerns, you may want to go to a therapist or counsellor who focuses on these topics.

Talking To Loved Ones

Talking to loved ones is a crucial aspect of self-care for males, as it supports mental and emotional health. Cultural expectations often encourage men to suppress their emotions, but maintaining open communication can offer numerous benefits.

It can provide emotional release, strengthen relationships and aid in problem-solving. Sharing thoughts and concerns with family members can lead to new insights and possible solutions. Regular communication with loved ones can help reduce loneliness and isolation, as they remind individuals they are not alone in dealing with life's challenges.

Regular communication also aids in the development of emotional resilience, enabling better stress management.

Suppressing feelings can exacerbate mental health problems like anxiety and sadness. Talking to loved ones can help manage and avoid these illnesses. Effective communication skills can be improved through conversations with close friends and family members. Setting an example by being honest about one's feelings and experiences can set a positive example for others, even younger generations. Progress in society depends on dismantling gender norms and promoting emotional expressiveness.

To get the greatest benefit from family conversations for self-care:

Choose the Right People: Look for people who are encouraging, understanding, and non-judgmental. They should be folks you feel at ease and trust.

Make a Safe Space by creating a setting that encourages direct and honest dialogue. Confidentiality and privacy are essential.

Be Vulnerable: Even if sharing your actual sentiments makes you feel exposed, do it nonetheless. Deeper relationships might result from being authentic in your communication.

Actively listening: Always keep in mind that communication is two-way. Pay attention to what your family members are saying and be there for them in the same way that they are there for you.

When necessary, seek professional assistance. If you have trouble opening up or are coping with complicated emotional problems, you may want to go to a therapist or counsellor. They may provide knowledgeable direction and assistance.

Finding Your Voice

Men's self-care includes finding their voices, which is crucial. It involves assertively and honestly expressing your opinions, feelings, and demands.

To find your voice, take time to reflect on your emotions and ideas, recognizing your values, opinions and feelings. Develop emotional intelligence by journaling and using active listening techniques when conversing. Seek help from friends, family or a therapist to share your worries and find your voice.

Establish limits in personal and professional life and assert them when needed. Practice assertiveness, expressing yourself while respecting others' needs and emotions.

Invest in hobbies and interests to express yourself creatively. Maintain physical well-being through regular exercise, a healthy diet and sufficient sleep, which can also influence emotional well-being. Meditation and mindfulness techniques can help communicate your feelings honestly.

Dispel prevailing masculine preconceptions that restrict emotional expressiveness and accept that it's okay to be open and seek assistance when necessary. Self-compassion is essential for self-care and should be understood and sympathetic to oneself. Study conflict resolution skills, paying attention actively, showing empathy and coming up with solutions that benefit all parties.

Spend time with supportive people who will support and encourage you while seeking your voice. A solid support network can significantly impact outcomes. Consistency in engaging in self-care and self-expression is essential, as it may take time and setbacks may occur.

PART 7: FROM DEPRESSION TO RESILIENCE

<u>Recognizing Signs Of Depression</u>

For early intervention and getting the right support, it's essential to recognise the symptoms of depression in yourself or another person. Depression is a significant mental health disease that has an impact on emotions, thinking and physical health.

Following are typical depression warning signs and symptoms:

Having a constant sense of sadness, emptiness or hopelessness, often for no apparent cause.

Loss of Interest: A decline in enjoyment or interest in past-time pursuits or hobbies.

Fatigue and Low Energy: Constantly feeling exhausted, even after a full night of sleep, and lacking the energy to do daily duties.

Alterations in sleep patterns, such as chronic insomnia *(difficulty getting or staying asleep)* or hypersomnia *(consistent oversleeping).*

Weight Changes or Appetite Changes: Significant changes in appetite might result in weight gain or reduction. Others may have diminished appetites, while others may overeat.

Irritability and Restlessness: Feeling easily agitated, nervous or annoyed without a known reason why.

Finding it hard to focus, make judgements or recall information. The results of job or academic work may be impacted.

Sentiments of Excessive Guilt or Worthlessness: Having excessive guilt or worthlessness sentiments, even when there is no justifiable reason for them.

Undiagnosed health complaints, such as headaches or stomach issues, that don't improve with therapy.

Withdrawal from friends, family and other social interactions. isolation and avoiding contact with others.

Suicidal Thoughts: Having thoughts of ending one's life via self-harm or another means. Speak with a mental health professional right away or call a crisis hotline if you or someone you know is having suicide thoughts.

Aches and Pains: Experiencing bodily symptoms such as aches, pains and digestive problems without a diagnosable underlying medical illness.

Not everyone will experience depression in the same way or display all of these symptoms. Also variable are the symptoms' intensity and duration. Others may have recurrent bouts of depression throughout the course of their life, while other individuals may only ever suffer one depressed episode.

Strategies For Coping With Depression

Seeking professional assistance from a mental health professional is essential if you or someone you know is dealing with depression. These tactics might be used in addition to professional treatment:

Seek expert assistance: A mental health professional, such a therapist, psychiatrist or counsellor, may provide direction, support, and treatment alternatives suited to your unique need.

Medication: For some people with depression, a psychiatrist's prescription medication may be a crucial component of their treatment strategy. To ascertain if a medicine is right for you, be sure to speak with a healthcare professional.

Psychotherapy: Various therapies, such as cognitive-behavioural therapy *(CBT)*, dialectical behaviour therapy *(DBT)*, or interpersonal therapy *(IPT)*, may assist people in developing coping mechanisms, challenging unhelpful thinking patterns and addressing underlying problems that contribute to depression.

Lean on your support network of friends and family for emotional assistance. Sharing your sentiments with others may boost your sense of community and make you feel less alone.

Join an advocacy group: You may meet others who are going through comparable difficulties via support groups, whether they are in person or online. It may be reassuring and beneficial to discuss struggles and coping mechanisms.

It's important to look after your mental and emotional well. This entails engaging in regular exercise, maintaining a healthy diet, giving sleep first priority and abstaining from alcohol and other drugs. Giving your day structure might help you feel more secure and purposeful. To feel successful, make tiny, attainable objectives for yourself.

You may regulate your stress and lessen the effects of unfavourable thoughts by engaging in mindfulness and meditation practices.

Avoid solitude by making an effort to contact others, even in little doses. Depression may cause you to desire to retreat from social activities. Over time, socialising might elevate your mood.

To reduce feelings of worry and overload, try stress-reduction exercises like deep breathing, progressive muscle relaxation or yoga. Also use approaches like cognitive restructuring to identify and confront negative thinking patterns. Replace unbalanced and unrealistic thinking with more sensible ones.

Set attainable objectives and divide larger activities into more manageable chunks. Your drive and self-worth might increase when you accomplish even modest objectives. Be sure to recognise and reduce exposure to people, places or circumstances that exacerbate your depressive symptoms.

Keep a diary, take part in artistic endeavours or find another productive method to communicate your feelings and ideas.

Be patient with yourself since depression recovery takes time and relapses are frequent. Recognise your progress, no matter how minor it may appear and have compassion for yourself.

There is no one-size-fits-all strategy for dealing with depression since it is a complicated disorder. Working with a healthcare practitioner to create a specialised treatment plan that takes into account your particular requirements and circumstances is important.

Seek urgent assistance from a mental health crisis hotline or a healthcare professional if you or someone you know is suffering from severe depression or is having thoughts of self-harm or suicide.

<u>Seeking Professional Help</u>

Reach out to trained specialists who can provide the right assistance and treatment since depression is a severe medical illness that may significantly affect your life.

Prior to getting assistance, it's critical to recognise the symptoms and indications of depression. These include feelings of despondency, lack of interest in previously enjoyed activities, changes in diet or sleep habits and more. It's important to pay attention to these signs if you or someone you know is exhibiting them.

Consult with your primary care doctor or general practitioner as a starting point. They may evaluate your symptoms, rule out any underlying illnesses, and provide therapy suggestions. They could suggest a mental health professional as well.

Depression may be diagnosed and treated by a mental health professional, such as a licensed therapist, psychiatrist or psychologist. Depending on your particular requirements, they may provide counselling, medicine or a mix of the two. By using your insurance provider, web directories or your healthcare provider, you may locate mental health providers.

Different forms of treatment and counselling may be helpful for depression. Some popular methods include dialectical behaviour therapy, interpersonal therapy and cognitive-behavioural therapy. You may acquire coping mechanisms, confront unhelpful thinking patterns and build better emotional regulation skills with therapy's assistance.

Psychiatrists are medical professionals who may write prescriptions and supervise patients' continuing pharmaceutical regimens. Taking medication may be helpful, particularly when combined with treatment.

Becoming a member of a support group for depression may provide you emotional support and a feeling of belonging. Sharing experiences with others who are facing comparable difficulties may be helpful and comforting.

Consider online treatment platforms that provide counselling and therapy sessions through video chat or texting if you have trouble getting to in-person therapy. These platforms may be practical and useful.

Please call for assistance right away if you're in crisis, having suicidal or self-harm ideas or if you think someone else could be in urgent danger. Visit the closest emergency hospital, dial a crisis hotline or contact emergency services.

Patience and consistency are vital throughout the course of depression treatment since it might take some time. Attend therapy sessions as scheduled, take prescription medicines exactly as instructed and be honest with your mental health professional about your progress and any difficulties you encounter.

Adopting a healthy lifestyle may help manage depression in addition to receiving expert therapy. This involves using stress-reduction strategies, eating a healthy diet and engaging in regular exercise.

Getting treatment for depression is a show of strength, not weakness. The support and direction you need to get through this difficult time and move towards recovery are things that mental health experts are equipped to provide.

Building Emotional Resilience

Emotional resilience is the ability to adapt and recover from life's challenges and disappointments. It involves controlling emotions, maintaining a positive attitude and handling stress effectively.

Techniques to develop emotional resilience include self-awareness, cultivating a growth mentality, using mindfulness practices like meditation and deep breathing exercises, creating a network of support, setting attainable goals, maintaining a healthy lifestyle, developing problem-solving abilities and developing optimism.

Self-awareness involves recognizing one's feelings and their causes, while a growth mentality accepts obstacles and failures as opportunities for improvement.
Mindfulness practices like meditation and deep breathing exercises help maintain presentness and grounding. Establishing close bonds with loved ones can provide emotional support when needed.

Maintaining a healthy lifestyle, such as eating a balanced diet, exercising regularly and sleeping adequately, also plays a significant role in emotional well-being. Focusing on solutions rather than issues can help develop problem-solving abilities.

Developing optimism involves admitting unpleasant feelings and seeking positive aspects for development. Controlling stress through effective strategies like time management, relaxation methods and establishing boundaries between personal and professional lives can help manage stress. Seeking professional assistance, practising self-compassion and learning to recognize and control emotions are essential for emotional resilience.

Embracing change as a natural part of life allows individuals to be more flexible and adaptive, better equipped to face unforeseen obstacles. By implementing these techniques, individuals can become more emotionally resilient and successful in their lives.

Developing emotional toughness is a continuous process. Time and practice are necessary. Be gentle with yourself and keep using these techniques to build emotional resilience and strength over time.

PART 8: BALANCING WORK AND LIFE

Setting Boundaries

It promotes stress reduction, a good work-life balance and general wellbeing. Here are some advice for males alone on how to create and maintain these boundaries:

Set Up a Clear Work Schedule:

Clearly define the beginning and finish of your workday. As you would if you were working in an office, try to adhere to these hours as precisely as you can.

Make a Specialised Workspace:

If you work from home, set aside a space only for that purpose. This makes it easier for you to cognitively distinguish between your personal and business spaces.

Clearly State boundaries:

Make sure everyone knows how important it is to respect your working hours, including your employer, coworkers and family. When you are available for work-related concerns and when you are not, be sure to make that clear.

Place Limits on Technology:

During your off-work hours, disable any emails or alerts relating to your job. By doing this, work won't interfere with your leisure time.

Personal Time Schedule:

Plan frequent breaks and time for recreation during your off-work hours. This might be resting, engaging in hobbies or engaging in physical activity.

Put self-care first:

Realise the importance of self-care for your physical and emotional health. Make time for rejuvenating hobbies like reading, meditation and lengthy baths.

Routine Exercise:

Working out is a fantastic technique to lower stress and boost your mood in general. Make frequent outdoor activities or exercises a part of your regimen.

Use relaxation and mindfulness techniques:

You may control your stress and maintain your equilibrium by using methods like yoga, deep breathing exercises and meditation.

Set Long-term Objectives:

Think about your long-term professional and personal objectives. Making choices regarding your employment that are in line with your larger life goals might be facilitated by having a clear vision.

Look for Support and Direction:

If you're having trouble setting or maintaining boundaries, don't be afraid to ask friends, family or a therapist for help. They may provide insightful advice and motivation.

How to Say No:

It's crucial to be forceful and to refuse requests when required. Overcommitting at work may have a detrimental effect on your personal life and cause burnout.

Consider and Correct:

Review your work-life balance often and make changes as necessary. Be willing to adjust your limits as necessary since life's circumstances change.

Establishing boundaries is a continuous process of which self-awareness and self-control are needed. You may achieve a healthy balance between your professional and personal life by prioritising your health and putting these techniques into practice, which will eventually improve your self-care as a man.

Time Management

Achieving a work-life balance is mandatory for long-term success and overall well-being. Effective time management techniques can help achieve this balance. To set specific priorities and goals, establish a schedule, block time, use to-do lists, establish limits, reduce distractions, collaborate and delegate, say no when necessary, get fresh air and prioritise self-care.

Create a schedule that includes work, personal life and self-care in your daily or weekly plan. Avoid multitasking and use productivity tools to maintain attention. Collaborate and delegate tasks to reduce workload and increase productivity. Say no when necessary to avoid overcommitting.

Incorporate rest intervals throughout working hours, such as stretching, meditation or engaging in fun activities. Prioritise self-care by setting aside time for leisure pursuits, exercise and other self-care activities.

Be adaptable and flexible with your schedule, as life is dynamic. Review and modify your time management techniques periodically to ensure their effectiveness.

Seek guidance from mentors, coaches or therapists if needed. Acknowledge and celebrate your successes in both professional and personal life to maintain equilibrium and also schedule quality time with family or friends to maximise personal life moments.

It may be difficult to find the ideal balance between work and life, and it may differ based on your circumstances and personal preferences. To create a balance that works best for you, it's important to continuously evaluate and modify your strategy.

Achieving Work-Life Harmony

To preserve their physical and mental health, reduce stress and enhance their overall quality of life, men must achieve a work-life balance. In order to do this, men should create clear boundaries between their personal and professional lives, set specific work hours, block off time for work-related tasks and emails, prioritise self-care, use effective time management techniques, assign tasks and refuse them.

Work shrewdly rather than hard, organise and plan, manage technology, engage in regular physical activity, seek help for mental health issues, spend meaningful time with family and friends, including things of interest.

Finally, men should be adaptable and flexible the way they communicate their priorities and limitations to their families, colleagues and employers.

Men may better manage their personal and professional lives and maintain a good work-life balance by adhering to these rules and giving self-care importance.

Please note that achieving work-life balance demands patience, self-awareness, restraint and commitment to one's well-being.

PART 9: CONCLUSION - A NEW PATH FORWARD

The Road To Well-Being

The process of a guy being happy is intricate and encompasses many facets of his social, emotional, mental and physical well-being. Men should strive for 7-9 hours of sleep each night, participate in regular physical exercise, and maintain a healthy diet to attain wellbeing.

Learn stress-reduction techniques such as yoga, deep breathing, mindfulness and meditation. When coping with mental health conditions like anxiety, melancholy or mood disorders, seek professional treatment. To cultivate a positive mindset, engage in acts of appreciation and challenge negative thought patterns.

Create emotional intelligence through identifying and comprehending one's own feelings as well as those of others in order to maintain psychological wellness. Develop healthy coping mechanisms and find outlets for your feelings, such as via hobbies, writing, art or chats with friends.

Maintain ties with friends and family by communicating and seeking out social support. Joining clubs may help you increase your social network and engage in the things you like.

Set short- and long-term goals for your career, personal development, and relationships with others. Create your objectives and engage in things that give your life meaning and purpose.

Prioritise your personal health, use time effectively to spread out duties and minimise stress to maintain a healthy work-life balance. To secure financial security in the future, establish a budget, save money and make smart investment decisions.

Being knowledgeable about personal finance can help you make informed choices regarding your money. Learn new things often, broaden your skill set and strive for both personal and professional progress.

Encouraging Change In Men's Lives

Promoting good change in men's life is great for individual development, improved interpersonal interactions and more cohesive societies.

Promoting open communication, raising mental health awareness, organising education and awareness campaigns, showcasing positive male role models, creating support groups, establishing mentoring programmes, supporting fatherhood initiatives, providing life skills training, career development, community engagement, counselling and therapy and advocating for policies and initiatives that promote gender equality are all strategies for encouraging change.

Men are better able to communicate their ideas, opinions and worries when there is open communication because they may do so without fear of repercussions. Mental health education spreads knowledge about the value of mental health and the need for resources and support systems.

Change is sparked by admirable role models who exhibit traits like empathy, vulnerability and emotional intelligence. While mentorship programmes combine seasoned men with those seeking advice, support groups provide men a forum to interact with others going through similar struggles.

While fatherhood programmes emphasise responsible parenting and the provision of tools for men to forge close ties with their children, promoting healthy relationships entails education and communication training.

Training in life skills, professional advancement, involvement in the community, counselling and treatment, advocacy and acknowledging accomplishments are all crucial tactics for encouraging good change in men's lives.

The Future Of Men's Mental Health

Men's mental health in the future is a crucial and developing subject that includes numerous facets of emotional health, masculinity and cultural developments.

Important factors for men's mental health in the future:

Destigmatization: In recent years, there has been an increased attempt to reduce the stigma associated with men's mental health difficulties. With more awareness efforts and conversations encouraging men to ask for assistance when necessary without feeling weak or humiliated, this trend is likely to continue.

Services for mental health that are more gender-responsive will be provided, taking into account that men may have different needs and preferences when it comes to getting support. This can include providing therapy groups with a male emphasis, online counselling services and specialised treatment plans.

Holistic methods: Men's mental health will move in the future towards more holistic methods. Along with conventional treatment and medicine, this entails taking into account how lifestyle elements like nutrition, exercise, sleep, and social relationships may have an influence.

Employers are becoming more aware of the value of assisting workers with their mental health in the workplace. With more businesses creating mental health programmes and providing resources to address workplace stress and mental health issues, this is expected to continue to expand.

Digital mental health: Technology will increasingly be used to assist mental health. Men will have simple and quick ways to monitor their mental health thanks to apps, internet resources and teletherapy services.

Cultural shifts: Men's mental health will be significantly impacted by societal changes in how masculinity is seen and defined. Men may feel more at ease expressing their feelings and requesting assistance when required when outdated notions about masculinity change.

Preventive Actions: To advance men's mental health, preventive action will get more attention. Programmes for early intervention in schools, public awareness campaigns and resources to assist men in identifying and managing stress and emotional difficulties before they worsen are included in this.

Peer support groups and men's support networks will probably become more and more popular. These provide men private locations where they may talk openly about their mental health issues, exchange stories, and encourage one another.

Data and Research: Ongoing research will make it possible to pinpoint the precise mental health conditions that disproportionately impact males. Interventions and treatments will become increasingly specialised as a result of this understanding.

Cultural Sensitivity: To better understand and manage the specific mental health needs of varied groups of men, taking into consideration aspects like race, ethnicity, and sexual orientation, mental health professionals will continue to focus on cultural sensitivity training.

TO EVERY MAN OUT THERE:

**YOUR ARE BRAVE, YOUR ARE STRONG
Most of all - YOU ARE HUMAN.**

GUIDE TO CREATING YOUR SELF-CARE WORKSHEET/PLAN

Self-Reflection:

- Write down three things that have been causing you stress or anxiety recently.
-
- Reflect on how these stressors make you feel emotionally and physically.

Self-Care Goals:

List three self-care goals you'd like to achieve in the near future. Make sure these goals are specific, achievable and time-bound.

Daily Self-Care Checklist:

Create a checklist with activities you want to do daily for self-care. Include items like:

- ☐ Meditation or deep breathing exercises.
- ☐ Physical activity *(e.g., exercise, yoga, stretching)*.
- ☐ Healthy eating *(e.g., balanced meals, drinking enough water)*.
- ☐ Quality sleep *(aim for 7-9 hours)*.
- ☐ Positive affirmations for gratitude journaling.
- ☐ Connect with a loved one *(e.g., call or meet up)*.
- ☐ Take breaks and practice mindfulness.
- ☐ Pursue a hobby or interest.

Weekly Self-Care Plan:

Outline your self-care activities for the upcoming week.
Assign specific days and times to each activity.

Self-Care Journal:

Use this section to jot down your thoughts and feelings after
practising self-care activities.

- Note any improvements in your mood, stress levels, or
  overall well-being.

Self-Care Rewards:

- List rewards or treats you can give yourself for achieving
  your self-care goals.

- These rewards can motivate you to prioritise self-care.

Emergency Self-Care Plan:

- Create a list of quick and easy self-care activities you can
  turn to when you're feeling overwhelmed.

- Include activities that can be done in 5-10 minutes.

Self-Care Support Network:

Write down the names and contact information of people you can
reach out to when you need support or someone to talk to.

Self-Care Affirmations:

- Write down positive affirmations or encouraging statements that resonate with you.
-
- Use them as reminders to practise self-compassion and self-care.

Progress Tracker:

- Use this section to track your progress in achieving your self-care goals over time.

- Note any challenges you face and how you overcome them.

Take Care & Be Healthy!

●

www.ingramcontent.com/pod-product-compliance
Lightning Source LLC
Chambersburg PA
CBHW050848260726

48660CB00006B/2516